*The*
# High Energy Diet
*Recipe Guide*

By
Dr. Douglas N. Graham

*The*
# High Energy Diet
*Recipe Guide*

2003

Inquiries regarding requests to reprint all or part of
*The High Energy Diet Recipe Guide* should be addressed to:

Dr. Douglas N. Graham
609 N. Jade Drive
Key Largo, FL 33037

phone: 305-852-0214
fax: 305-852-0215
email: foodnsport@aol.com
www.doctorgraham.cc

# Dedication

This book is dedicated to two super achievers—my best teachers, my loving parents, Marty and Bea. Your constant love, encouragement, and support have allowed me to grow into the person that I am today. I have attempted to learn as much as possible from you, to incorporate the best from both of you into my personality and pass it on to others, to learn from your mistakes.

I hope that I can surpass your highest dreams for me, and that the recipes in this book will bring you great enjoyment and long-lasting health.

# Acknowledgments

Helping people to achieve their goals brings me tremendous satisfaction. There are many people who should have the feeling of satisfaction about my completing this book, without whose support it could never have been done. They are, indeed, too numerous to name individually.

Every staff member has shielded me, allowing me to sit and write rather than be interrupted or distracted; thank you. Every hygienic professional, those who led before me as well as my colleagues, have motivated me with their unfailing examples of service and achievement.

Thank you, Shari, for being so understanding, for realizing that producing this book was, for me, a mission. Thank you for handling virtually everything else while this project held my full attention.

Special thanks to Laurie Masters, whose extraordinary editing skills and reliability with every detail made this book possible and readable.

Thank you to everyone who has encouraged me to finish this project: patients, family, and friends. If hundreds of you had not demanded it, again and again, I am sure I would never have written it.

# Table of Contents

# Preface

If they'd needed a cookbook in Eden, this could have been the one, full of heavenly delicacies from the orchard and garden. This is euphoria food; too-good-to-be-good-for-you food; succulent, flavorful, exquisite food. The fact that it also has the ability to ensure and even restore a high level of health and vitality comes about because this is not so much a cookbook as a cook-less book: Not one of the glorious recipes on its pages requires a stove, oven, or microwave, just a working relationship with your local greengrocer.

Adding more fresh, uncooked foods to your diet is a treat that can also be a challenge. We need help in trading in old habits for better ones, and the beautiful, easy-to-prepare recipes on these pages provide that help deliciously.

Most of us were brought up on heavy foods, cooked and overcooked, with animal products on center stage and refined sweets and snack foods playing major supporting roles. We're better educated today and are planning meals with lower cholesterol and lower overall fat levels, more fiber, and fewer unnecessary chemical additives. These are major steps in the direction of lifetime health and nonstop energy. In The High Energy Diet Recipe Guide however, Dr. Graham takes us even further, to a way of eating that supplies us with all the vital force of natural foods, straight from the earth to the table.

As a longtime health writer, I have learned about numerous dietary philosophies. I have seen that any change from the burger-and-fries norm brings about noticeable improvement in the life of the person who tries it.

For this reason, I applaud those who are sharing with us ways to cut the fat in our cooking methods, those who encourage a gradual shift to a more vegetarian diet, the macrobiotic community, and those in medicine and dietetics who challenge the traditional Four Foods Groups and are providing the public with better choices.

The choice offered by Dr. Graham is, in my opinion, optimal. I base this not only on research and interviews with experts over the years, but on my own experience. I always eat "well", That is, I am a complete vegetarian; I do not eat fried foods or sugary, salty snack foods; I don't drink coffee or colas. Nevertheless, there are times when my vitality lags, when I don't feel infused with life first thing in the morning. Those are the times I need to remind myself to increase the fresh, uncooked fruits, vegetables and juices in my diet. When I do this, I bounce back in just a day or two—the was a droopy, dry houseplant perks up after a good watering.

Dr. Graham's recipes are just what the doctor ordered for keeping the level of fresh, unprocessed foods high in my diet and yours. Colorful fruits and vegetables are bursting with vitamins, minerals, and enzymes that cooking destroys in short order. The raw nuts and seeds used moderately in some of the recipes provide satiety and essential fatty acids without resorting to extracted oils or heated fats that are believed to have carcinogenic properties.

In addition to these physical benefits, featuring uncooked foods as the predominant part of your diet offers more subtle rewards as well: you'll spend less time in the kitchen; you'll have more hours for exercise, relaxation, expanding your mind, enjoying your hobbies, and being with those you love.

Be gentle with yourself as you embark upon this new adventure. It isn't all or nothing. It is instead a process of growth: try at least one of these recipes every day for a month. See what happens. See how you feel. Listen to your body. Trust it. Go with the seasons as they change. And remember that life produces life: the more living foods you include in your daily menus, the more living you are apt to pack into every day. And thanks to Dr. Graham, you can do this eating "fudge" and "chocolate pudding."

Victoria Moran
Author, *The Love-Powered Diet*

# Foreword

Welcome to *The High Energy Diet Recipe Guide*. Using diet in the sense that what you eat is your diet, *The High Energy Diet* will provide you with ideas for the ultimate in healthy eating. Whether you have been a long time purist or this is your first experiment with improving your food regime, *The High Energy Diet* will help you to make great strides.

The outstanding feature of this book is that all the recipes are prepared from 100 per cent raw foods. This is not to say that I think cooking is to be wholly avoided, more that I feel the reader is already competent in the art of creating cooked food dishes. This effort is geared towards helping you create healthy raw food recipes which I hope will eventually become the mainstay of your diet. As you add in more uncooked meals you will become fluent with the art of developing them on your own. Your overall percentage of uncooked foods will increase. I am striving to help you achieve a diet characterized by an abundance of raw foods in which fruits and vegetables predominate. This type of diet is universally accepted as one which will help you to reach your fullest health potential while doing yourself and the environment the least possible harm.

I have tried to be as specific as possible with this Guide. However, I encourage you to experiment, substitute, and find out just exactly what best fits your needs and satisfies your tastes. There is always room for questions. I appreciate your questions, comments, and feedback. Please let me know if you found this booklet useful, or how you think I could improve upon it. It is my sincerest wish that you will find this book and its audio and video companions of immense value.

# The Advantages of a Raw-Food Diet

The concept of this book is simple: to help you incorporate more uncooked recipes into your yearly meal plan. With practice you will become talented in serving raw-food dishes. As you increase your creativity and ability to make them delicious for you and your loved ones, you will find that eating garden-fresh food is really most satisfying.

The most obvious advantage of a raw-food diet is that every meal is *quick to prepare*. That is not to say that you can't prepare complex and fascinating meals, but rather you have the chance for each meal to be zero prep. Think of the time you usually spend in the kitchen preparing your average dinner. Compare that to a meal of watermelon. Bacon and eggs, pancakes, even a simple sandwich, all take preparation time that makes fruit look like the original "fast food."

To ensure that you get the absolute maximum in *nutritional density*, your foods must be eaten in a raw state with as little preparation as possible. Heat is one of the main destroyers of nutrients in your food. Enzymatic destruction begins at 116 degrees; vitamins lose potency at 130 degrees; and proteins become denatured above 161 degrees Fahrenheit. (Denatured proteins are unusable to your body, cannot be "renatured," and have been linked with many diseases, including arthritis, heart disease and even cancer.) Try sticking your hand in boiling water for even a moment if you want to see proteins denatured. Even steaming vegetables requires a temperature of 212 degrees. While heated foods will deliver caloric density more easily than their raw counterparts, most of the nutrients have been cooked out.

If you are looking for calories without nutrients, cooked foods are the best source. If you want the highest possible nutrient count per calorie, eat raw foods.

Perhaps the most noticeable feature of a raw meal is that it is so incredibly *easy to clean up*. Greases are almost never present, and nothing is ever baked onto the pan or dish. Usually all it takes to clean up is a quick rinse with water only. Sometimes a sponge is necessary to remove a spot of nut butter or a sticky bit of fruit.

When you eat raw foods you can guarantee that your meals will be *always fresh*. Did you ever hear of someone giving themselves food poisoning on fresh fruit? Of course not, because when the food is raw, it is easy to tell if it has gone "bad." Fresh whole raw fruits and vegetables are rich in color, flavor, and textures, too.

Perhaps the most important reason for eating a predominantly raw food diet is that it is *environmentally responsible*. No packaging need be manufactured or thrown away. Energy is not required to heat the food. Rain forests are saved rather than cut to raise livestock. Animals are nurtured, not destroyed. With more than 50 percent of our nation's water supply and 80 percent of our grains going to raise livestock, a diet high in fruits and vegetables is environmentally sound.

I sincerely hope that you will find the recipes in this book as delicious and easy to prepare as I do. I look forward to receiving your comments and suggestions. Enjoy your meals.

In Abundant Health,
Dr. Douglas N. Graham

# COLD SLAWS

Shred a vegetable and you have a slaw. Slaws are one of my favorite vegetable meals, because they are easy to eat and have potential for so much variety. The mechanical digestion has been partially done by machines, making slaws a good choice for people with chewing difficulties or for people who are not yet used to the amount of chewing necessary for a fresh, vegetable meal.

# CASHEW SLAW

Grate:    1/2 head green cabbage
          1/4 head red cabbage
          6 celery stalks
          1 large red bell pepper

Top with 4 to 8 ounces of Cashew Cream (p. 13) and mix thoroughly.

Optional: Sprinkle lightly with powdered caraway seed.

# CAUL SLAW

Shred:    1 head cauliflower
          1 medium bunch celery.
Blend:    High, for one minute.
          8 ounces soaked, blanched raw almonds
          with 4 ounces water.

Blend in 4 ounces of fresh squeezed orange juice for a sweet dressing, plus the juice of one lemon or lime if you prefer a "bite."

Mix all the ingredients with the dressing.

Add in 4 diced tomatoes.

# CELERY SLAW

| Grate: | 1 large bunch celery |
|---|---|
| | 2 red bell peppers |
| Blend: | 3 or 4 tomatoes |
| | 4 ounces walnuts |
| | Makes a dressing. |

Mix all the ingredients with the dressing.

Serve lemon on the side.

# GREEN SLAW

| Shred: | 1/2 head green cabbage |
|---|---|
| | 1 medium bunch of celery |
| Blend: | 2 avocados |
| | 1 stalk of broccoli |
| | 8 ounces water |
| | Makes a dressing. |

Mix all the ingredients with the dressing.

Garnish by thinly slicing one red bell pepper onto the top.

# SPROUT SLAW

Chop:         2 four-ounce containers of alfalfa sprouts
into half-inch lengths
Mix in:      1/2 pound mung bean sprouts
Shred:      1/4 head  green cabbage
Blend:      2 avocados with 4 tomatoes
Pour this over vegetables.

Mix and serve garnished with whole celery stalks.

# RED SLAW

Shred:      1/2 head red cabbage
2 cucumbers
Blend:      6 to 8 tomatoes
4 ounces of pecans
Makes a dressing.

Optional:   1 tablespoon dehydrated beet powder

Pour dressing over shredded vegetables.

Mix and serve.

# SUPER SALADS

Salads make up a big part of, and sometimes our entire, dinner meal almost every evening. I have found that there is much more room for variety, night after night, if I keep down the number of ingredients in each salad. Here are some of my tried-and-true favorites, but in reality I make a different salad every time.

# GREEK SALAD

Mix:        2 diced tomatoes
            1 diced zucchini
            8 ounces of mung bean sprouts
            (or other nonstarchy sprouts)
            1 finely chopped red pepper
            1 cup chopped, young okra

Blend:      12 black olives
            2–4 ounces water
            Makes a dressing.

Recommended: Rinse and soak olives for several hours, changing the water hourly, to remove brine.

## ITALIAN SALAD, SOUTHERN STYLE

Break:      1 bunch broccoli
            1 half head cauliflower
Chop:       1 romaine lettuce
            1 pound whole green olives
Blend:      4 or more dried tomatoes
            1 pint of water (to rehydrate)
            8  fresh basil leaves
            Makes a dressing.

Serve dressing on the side.

# EGGLESS SALAD

Grate:     1 yellow summer squash
           1 cucumber
           4 celery stalks
           1/4 head green cabbage

Serve on a bed of romaine lettuce.

Optional: Add whipped avocado, pine nuts, sprouted garbanzos or diced white mild radish.

# CLASSIC TOMATO SALAD

Dice:     4 tomatoes
          1 avocado

Toss well, mound on a bed of leaf lettuce and place 1 or 2 thinly sliced cucumbers around tomato avocado mix.

Cover lightly with grated red and green cabbage.

Optional: Add any mild herb. Each one creates a whole new salad.

# GREEN "KEYS" SALAD

Chop:        Broccoli
Leaf lettuce
Celery
Sprouts
Tomatoes

Mix with the blended milk and meat of 1 coconut.

# BROCCOMOLE SALAD

Finely chop:  1 bunch raw broccoli
3 red bell peppers

Mix with 1 bunch of coarsely cut leaf lettuce.

Pour on 1 avocado blended with 1 key lime.

# CORN SALAD

Cut:          The kernels off 6 ears of fresh, sweet corn
Dice:         2 cucumbers
              1 medium bunch celery
Finely chop:  1 sprig parsley

Mix all ingredients.

Use herbs or dried vegetables sparingly to flavor.


# MACCABBAGE SALAD

Chop:    1 small head green cabbage
         1 small head romaine
Dice:    4 tomatoes
Blend:   4 ounces raw macadamias
         3 to 4 ounces water
         The juice of 1 lime
         Makes a dressing.

## LAYERED SALAD

On a bed of romaine or other greens, add layers of the following:

> Large sliced tomatoes
> Avocado
> Cucumber
> Red pepper rings
> Sprouts

Serve in a clear glass bowl.

## RAINBOW SALAD

Using a round platter place arcs of equal portions of the following grated vegetables:

> Beets
> Carrots
> Yellow squash
> Broccoli
> Red cabbage

Beets go on top, red cabbage is the innermost arc.

Blend:
> Yellow corn
> Avocado
> Yellow bell peppers
> Makes an excellent "pot of gold" dressing.

# TOPPINGS

Toppings, the most visible portion of any dish, all start the same way. Their names—sauces, dips, spreads, icings, fondues, jams—are derived from their intended use and consistency. The same recipe can be used as a topping for fruit ice cream, as a spread over fruit compote, or as an icing for fruit pies.

Most of my sweet sauces consist of one dried fruit blended with water. I make them for sweetness as well as color. I am especially fond of pineapple, (pale yellow) persimmon (red) carob (dark brown) raisin (dark) date (light brown) canistel (deep yellow) and mammea (pink).

Toppings tend to be a bit more concentrated in both flavor and calories. I use toppings to entice the eater by adding artistic flair, color, and taste. Have fun making toppings. Get good at it, for these finishing touches are what your dining guests will remember most.

# ORANGE AND WALNUT SAUCE

Soak 4 ounces of walnut for 12 to 24 hours.

Change the water several times, or the walnut sauce will be quite tart.

Blend:        High for 1 minute
Walnuts soaked in 4 ounces
freshly squeezed orange juice

# COCONUT PINEAPPLE ORANGE SAUCE

Blend:        1 pineapple
4 oranges
Meat and milk of 1 coconut

# COCONUT DIP WITH PEAR AND APPLE

Use the "S" blade of a food processor.

Mix:        Meat and milk of 1 coconut
2 pears
2 apples
4 stalks finely chopped celery

## ALMOND DIP WITH
## PINEAPPLE AND STRAWBERRY

Blend:        4 ounces raw, soaked blanched almonds
1 pineapple
1 pint strawberries

## CASHEW CREAM

Soak 4 ounces raw cashews (whole or pieces) for 4-24 hours in enough distilled water to cover completely.

Blend nuts and water on high for 1 minute, adding water a little at a time if necessary.

## SALSA

Use a blender or food processor.

Mix:        2 tomatoes
               4 tomatillos
               4 leaves basil
               2 leaves oregano
Mince:     1 cucumber
               1 red bell pepper
               2 inches mild Daikon radish

Pour mixed ingredients over minced ingredients.

Serve with vegetables.

# APPLE WALNUT GRAPE SPREAD

Blend:      4 ounces raw, soaked walnuts
Grate:      2 apples
Crush:      1 bunch concord or other dark grapes

Mix all ingredients lightly.


# PAPAYA SPREAD

Peel and deseed one large papaya.
Cut into 2- inch squares.

Slowly add into blender.
Add lime to taste.

You may also need a tiny bit of water depending on the papaya.

Optional: Add 1 pint strawberry or 1/2 pineapple.

# FRUIT FONDUE

Dice equal amounts of the following:
> Banana
> Mango
> Apple
> Pear

Arrange on a platter with toothpicks in each piece or with fondue forks.

Make 3 thick sauces (fondues):

> - Dates and water
> - Raisins and water
> - Dried pineapple and water

Put each sauce in a separate bowl and enjoy by dipping fruit into the sauce.

Serve with a platter of lettuce and celery.

# VEGETABLE FONDUE

Cut equal amounts of the following vegetables:
Broccoli
Cauliflower
Celery
Yellow bell pepper
Zucchini

Arrange them on a platter.

Using a food processor create 3 thick fondue sauces out of the following vegetables:

- Tomato, tomatillo, celery, dried beet powder
- Cucumber, basil, oregano, avocado
- Cabbage, corn, rosemary, red bell pepper

Serve with fondue forks or as finger food.

# NUTTY FONDUE

Create a platter of vegetables or a platter of "acid" fruit,

Use your food processor to mix the following three fondues out of nuts and water:

- Cashews and water
- Almonds and water
- Sesame and water

Serve in classic fondue style, with fondue forks.

# AVOCADO ICING

Blend 2 avocados until creamy, adding a little water if necessary.

Optional: blend in two stalks of celery.

## ANY NUT ICING

Place 4 ounces of any raw soaked nuts in the blender.
Add water slowly and blend to desired consistency.

Note: Nuts go in the blender first, but too many nuts may
burn out your blender. Start with 2 ounces of nuts then a
bit of water. Add 2 more ounces and a bit more water.
You're more likely to run out of nuts before you run out of
water, so put the nuts in first and add water as needed.

## YOUR BASIC JAM

Soak 8 ounces of dried fruit in an equal amount of water
for 8 hours.

Blend to desired consistency by adding a bit more water
or a bit more dried fruit.

## HAWAIIAN CRUSH

Blend:        1 ripe pineapple
               Juice of 6 oranges
               2 ounces nuts (your choice)

# FRUIT SOUPS

Fruit soups greatly broaden your scope of variety and presentation. They make a tasty first course to almost any meal and are great served as a complete meal. Many people find that they can consume fruit more easily as soup than in any other form, Enjoy these sweet soups on a hot summer night when you would rather be cool.

## MELON SOUP

Put a little melon into a blender and blend briefly. As soon as it liquefies, add more. Keep adding melon and blending till you have a blender full.

Blend your choice of 2 or 3 different cold melons. Serve thick or strain for a delicious summer treat.

## STRAWBERRY SOUP

Blend 2 quarts of fresh or frozen strawberries with a little water.

Separately blend 4 ounces soaked raw cashews and 2 to 4 ounces water.

Gently pour cashew mix in a swirl over strawberries.

Serve with thinly sliced strawberries floating on top.

## SWEET APPLE SOUP

Blend well:    4 large Delicious apple chunks and blend
1 cup soaked raisins
2 to 4 cups water
1 sapodilla

(If you can't find sapodilla use 1 pear and 1/4 teaspoon cinnamon.)

Stir in one grated apple.

Note: This may be too sweet for you. To reduce the sweetness, blend in 1/2 stalk celery for every apple.

## GRAPEFRUIT SOUP

Squeeze 1 quart of fresh pink grapefruit juice and serve in a bowl over 1 pint of the berry of your choice.

## GRAPE SOUP

Squeeze 1 pint of orange juice and 8 ounces of grapefruit juice.

Pour the citrus mixture over 3 or 4 dozen grapes (variety of your choice).

Optional: Use lychees, fresh or frozen, instead of grapes.

# JUST DESSERTS

Everybody has a sweet tooth. This is natural to us, so that we will reach for fruits to satisfy our need for fuel in the vitamin C complex. Fruits are the best source of almost every vitamin. When people ask, "But don't you like sweets?" they are showing that they don't understand how many sweets you really do eat.

It is easy to overeat on these sweet meals; take your time. When eating, include lettuce and/or celery with your sweet meals. Balance your sugar intake with your activities, and remember to always listen to your body.

## FUDGE S'MORES

Soak 1 pound dates and 6 ounces raisins in distilled water for 2 hours.

Layer dates, raisins, and Fruit Gellée (p. 42) into a square dish. Sprinkle lightly with raw carob powder.

Freeze and serve with lettuce.
Optional: cover with crushed nuts.

Note: this holiday treat can be a tough combination to digest.

## FUDGE

Using the "S" blade of a food processor, mix equal parts of date and banana. Process until completely smooth. You may need to add a few ounces of water, but add sparingly, as needed.

Finely dice 2 inches of vanilla bean and add to mixture.

Keep food processor running and slowly add 1–2 teaspoons raw carob powder to taste. If mix is not dry enough or you would like a more chewy consistency, add a few ounces of chopped, dried fruit.

Shape to desired form, freeze and serve. This fudge will not freeze solid.

Serve with lettuce and celery as a dessert after fruit or as a sweet fruit meal.

# MANGO DELIGHT

Dice 4 mangos into a bowl and squeeze on the juice of one lime.

This simple, delicious meal is tough to surpass.

# AMBROSIA

Blend:      1 bunch grapes
Grate:      2 tart apples

Mix:        Blended grapes
            Grated apples
            Milk and meat of 1 young coconut

Serve in a pie dish and top with sliced stone fruit .

# CITRUS AMBROSIA

Dice:       6 oranges
            2 grapefruits
            1 pineapple
            2 tangerines
            2 starfruit

Grate the meat of one ripe coconut.

Mix all ingredients including the milk of the coconut.

## JAM "HANDWICH"

Slice 1 very ripe banana lengthwise.
Place on 1 or 2 large leaves of romaine lettuce.

Spread banana with Your Basic Jam (p. 19).
Roll up the lettuce and serve as a "handwich."

## COOKIES

Using the food processor, mix:

> 4 ounces dried fruit
> 2 ripe bananas

Add water slowly as needed.

If desired, you may add minute amounts of minced ginger, raw carob powder, cocoa, or vanilla.

Form into balls, logs or discs. Roll in grated coconut and serve frozen on a large bed of lettuce.

Note: This can be a tough combination to digest. Enjoy some lettuce along with the cookies.

# DANDY CANDY

The variations on this basic recipe are endless.
Mix in any of the ingredients below using equal portions
of dry and moist ingredients to achieve a thick, gooey,
sticky consistency.

- Any chopped or ground nut or seed:
    Pecan, almond, walnut, sesame, etc.
- Dried fruit:
    Peaches, apples, prunes, figs, dates, papaya,
    mango, raisin, apricot, etc.
- Suitable spice:
    Cinnamon, ginger, carob, vanilla, nutmeg, cocoa
- Fresh fruit juice:
    Apple, lemon, orange, grape, grapefruit,
    cranberry, pineapple
- Nut butter:
    Macadamia, almond, sunflower, cashew, pistachio

Make cookies softer by adding mashed ripe banana.

Shape into the cookie shape of your choice.
Decorate with currants, raisins, or coconut.

Chili and serve.

# COOL SOUPS

Vegetable soups can be enjoyed as a complete meal or as a delicious dish early on in a multicourse meal. For people who find eating vegetables a chore, soups are an easy alternative. Soups make eating vegetables a pleasure. Vegetables are the number one source of virtually every mineral. Use vegetable soups to "use up" large amounts of many vegetables at once so that you don't ever have to deal with spoilage.

## GAZPACHO II

Blend:    6 tomatoes
              1 medium bunch celery

Pour over 4 ounces of finely chopped alfalfa sprouts.
Add 1 diced avocado if desired.

## BORSCHT

Peel, shred and blend:
              4 medium beets
              1 small bunch celery
              Milk of 1 young coconut
              8 ounces of water

Blend the meat of the coconut long enough and with sufficient water to make "cream."

Serve borscht in individual bowls and add "cream" separately.

## CUKE SOUP

Blend:    8 cucumbers
              4 ounces sesame tahini
              4 celery stalks

Add water as desired and pour over shredded cabbage.

# CREAMY GAZPACHO SOUP

Blend:        7 tomatoes
                4 ounces cashews (or cashew butter)

Dice:         2 red bell peppers
                8 celery stalks
                1 tomato

Pour soup over diced veggies and garnish with lime rounds.

# ASPARAGUS SOUP

Chop:        6 celery stalks
                4 ounces alfalfa sprouts

Crush:       4 ounces soaked, blanched almonds

Blend:       1 bunch of asparagus (not the tips)
                1 quart of water

Pour asparagus mixture over chopped vegetables.

Garnish with 1 thinly sliced yellow pepper and the asparagus tips.

# GAZPACHO SOUP

Blend:      8–10 tomatoes
Juice of 2 limes

Chop:      5 stalks celery
2 cucumbers
1 red bell pepper
1 orange bell pepper
1 yellow summer squash

Pour blended tomato over chopped vegetables.

Garnish lightly with sunflower seeds.

Serve slightly chilled.

# CLASSIC TOMATO CELERY SOUP

Use the "S" blade of a food processor to liquefy 4 tomatoes.

Cut 8 stalks of celery into 2-inch lengths and add them to the tomatoes.

Process briefly until the celery mixes in, but leave it slightly coarse.

Serve with lemon on the side.

31

# CREAMY TOMATO CELERY SOUP

Totally blend: 6–8 tomatoes
8 ounces cashews
6–8 celery stalks
1–2 pints water

Garnish with finely chopped ripe pineapple.

# CREAMY CORN SOUP

Blend: Kernels from 6 ears field-fresh sweet corn
2 cucumbers
1 pint water
1 avocado

Pour over 1/4 head finely chopped green cabbage, and chopped sprouts.

Garnish with a sprig of parsley.

# CAULIFLOWER SOUP

Blend:       1 cauliflower
              8 ounces pecans
              1 quart water

Finely chop:  1 bunch broccoli
              2 inches daikon radish
              1 bell pepper
              1 zucchini

Mix all ingredients and garnish around the edges with cauliflower and broccoli greens.

# PIES IN YOUR EYES

Who said eating simple fare needed to be boring? Anything but. Pies can be wholesome, delicious and beautiful; just use your imagination. Anything goes. Your delicious fruit pies will be talked about, and copied, every time you let your friends and family try them.

# HOLIDAY PIE

Use the "S" blade of a food processor.
Mix well:    1/2 pound honey dates
              4 ounces crushed walnuts

Layer in sliced fruit for color and flavor:
       -Strawberry, banana, blueberry, kiwi, apple.
Pour about 4 ounces of fresh fruit juice or blended fruit over sliced fruit.

Top with crushed coconut or nut butter dressing.
Decorate with sliced fruit. The variations are endless.
Use your imagination. Freeze and serve

Note: This pie can be tough to digest. Serve with plenty of celery and lettuce.


# SWEET MANGO PIE

Soak one pound of dates for one hour. Homogenize them in the food processor or Champion juicer with the blank plate.

Spread dates evenly onto a pie plate, up the sides and over the edges.

Run frozen mango through a Champion juicer with the blank plate to make mango ice cream and fill plate. Top decoratively with sliced banana. Freeze and serve.

# MANGO PIE

Soak 1 pound of pecans overnight.

Use the "S" blade of a food processor to reduce nuts to a "dough by slowly adding water. Spread dough into a pie plate up onto and over the sides.

Add even layers of strawberry and then mango ice cream (made in a Champion juicer with the blank plate).

Decorate around the perimeter with whole strawberries turned upside down.

Freeze and serve.

# FIGGY PIE

Cut off the stems and soak 24 blond calmyrna figs and 24 black mission figs.

Use the food processor to mix black figs with just enough water to make a "pie crust."

Fill crust with "Good Ol' Ice Cream" (p. 42), one layer of banana and one layer of peach. Make a top layer of blond figs.

Freeze and serve.

# CAROBANANA MINT PIE

Press a layer of pitted dates into the bottom of a glass pie dish.

Run frozen bananas through a Champion juicer with the blank plate. Layer into the pie dish about 3/4 inches thick.

Put this partially full dish into the freezer.

Run more bananas through the Champion and put them into a food processor.

Add 1 tablespoon raw carob powder and 1 tablespoon finely diced fresh mint leaves.

Mix for about 30 seconds or until bananas look completely dark.

Add this dark carob-mint-banana mix onto the top of the pie.

Decorate with 8 mint sprigs spaced evenly around the edge of the pie.
Freeze and serve.

## BERRY GOOD PIE

Use a Champion juicer with the blank plate.
Mix enough frozen strawberries to make a "crust."

Add a layer of blueberries and a layer of blackberries
Top with a layer of thinly sliced strawberries.

Blend:          Milk and meat of 1 coconut
                1/2 very ripe pineapple

Pour this mixture into the pie dish until it is full.
Decorate pie with an extra ring of raspberries.
Freeze and serve.


## ALL-AMERICAN PIE

Use a Champion juicer with the blank plate to make
**separate batches** of ice cream out of the following:
        4 peeled, frozen apples
        3 pints frozen strawberries
        1 pint frozen blueberries.

On a rectangular platter place alternating rows of frozen
apple and frozen strawberry to make stripes. Place the
frozen blueberry in a square in the top left corner.

Cut a fresh starfruit into 1/2-inch thick, star-shaped slices
and place them on and around the blue area of the pie.

# S'MORE JUST DESSERTS

Most people have the toughest time with lunch! Breakfast is easy: juicy fruit. Dinner is easy: lots of salad, vegetables, (raw and/or cooked) and a choice of starch, protein, or neither. But usually it is at lunch that the compromising begins. Salads are often unsatisfying, fruits don't hold you over. Have both! Enjoy sweet fruit lunches with plenty of lettuce and celery. Here's how.

## TROPICAL LUNCH

Dice 4 carambola (star fruit) into a bowl and cover with fresh 1queezed grapefruit juice.

Decorate with 1 sliced tangerine.

Serve with lettuce.

## FRUIT COMPOTE

Cut off the stems and blend 24 black or blond figs with enough water to make a runny sauce.

Shred 2 apples and 8 stalks of celery.

Mix all ingredients together and serve.

## FIGGY PUDDIN'

After cutting off the stems, soak 6 to 10 dried figs, any variety, overnight, using enough water to cover them completely.

Blend figs and their soak water.

Add water to reach desired consistency.

Serve with lettuce and celery.

# BANANA ICE CREAM

Peel and freeze fully ripe bananas.

Run uncut frozen bananas through Champion juicer. This procedure will work in a food processor; you just have to go a little slower. It will even work in a blender; just go slowly and add a little water as needed.

Serve immediately with lettuce.

# GLAZED STRAWBERRIES

Use the "S" blade of a food processor.

Mix:        2 ounces cold distilled water (approx.)
            4 ounces raw cashew butter

Mix until a thick creamy consistency is reached.

Cashew butter can be purchased raw at your health food store.

Dip fresh cold strawberries into cashew mix.
Serve with lettuce.

## GOOD OL' ICE CREAM

Run frozen fruit through a Champion using the blank.

Banana and other sweet fruits come out like soft ice cream. Subacid fruits come out like sherbet. Acid fruits and melon have the texture of Italian ices.

We prefer to eat the ice cream around the edges as it melts.

## CHICO PUDDING

This fruit is worth seeking out.
It can be ordered from fruit suppliers in south Florida. Fresh and raw, this fruit tastes similar to pears baked with cinnamon.

Mash 2 ripe skinned and deseeded sapodilla (chico) with a fork and serve.

Add over figgy puddin' or mashed banana for a real treat.

## BANANA SPLIT

Run 4 frozen bananas through the Champion juicer.

Add 3 scoops of ice cream to one "split" banana.

Pour on "Your Basic Jam" (p.19) of choice.

## FRUIT GELLÉE

Soak 4 ounces dried fruit in 8 ounces water.
Use the food processor to mix the fruit in just enough
water to mix.

Allow mixture to "set" for an hour or more in the
refrigerator. If it does not set, add a few chopped raisins
to soak up excess water.

Serve with lettuce and celery.

## COULD IT BE CHOCOLATE PUDDING?

Blend:      12 dates
               12 black mission figs
               1 quart water.
(More or less water may be needed depending on the
"dryness" of your fruit. Start with slightly less.)

Add 1 teaspoon of raw carob powder.

Chill and serve in pudding glasses.

# WHAT'S SHAKIN'

Shakes are the wholesome answer to the fast food question. Nutritionally complete, delicious, and easy to eat, shakes make a great meal in a glass or thermos. You will learn how much it takes to satisfy you and with very little practice become a shake master. Breakfast, lunch, or dinner, it is hard to beat a shake, especially if you don't have the time to luxuriate over a meal.

# TIPS FOR MAKING SHAKES

Start with your blender half full of water. Add a mixture of fresh and frozen fruit until you reach your desired flavor, sweetness, thickness and temperature. This will take practice hut is an art worth perfecting.

Note: Almost all thick sweet shakes contain banana. Strawberry, mango, orange, and other juicy fruit also make great shakes and tend to be less caloric, hence have less "staying" power. For those of you who find concentrated sugars give you trouble, or if you want to add more minerals to your diet, add in at least 1 stalk of celery for every 16 ounces of shake. It tastes great.

## CLASSIC SWEET SHAKES

Blend any of the following:

| | |
|---|---|
| banana, date | banana, water |
| banana, carob | banana, mango |
| banana, vanilla | banana, papaya |
| banana, raisin | banana, pineapple |
| banana, apple | banana, persimmon |
| banana, blueberry | banana, pear |

Feel free to experiment! Changing the amount of water, the number and or kind of fruit, or the temperature of the ingredients all change the meal dramatically. ENJOY!!

## PEACHBERRY SHAKE

Fill blender half full of water.

Add frozen peaches until almost full.

Top off with any berry.


## QUARTER SHAKE

Blend:          1/4 avocado
                1 quart of fresh-squeezed orange juice.

Add avocado to taste, but beware, too much avocado ruins this drink.


## TROPICAL DELIGHT

Blend:          Orange juice
                Papaya
                Pineapple

Add coconut to thicken.

# CLASSIC "JUICY" SHAKES

Blend any of the following:

| | |
|---|---|
| orange, berry | strawberry, grapefruit |
| orange, tomato | strawberry, mango |
| orange, plum | strawberry, peach |
| | |
| papaya, nectarine | pineapple, cherry |
| papaya, tangerine | pineapple, pear |
| papaya, passionfruit | pineapple, apple |

## FIVE-STAR SHAKE

Squeeze 1 pint fresh orange juice into the blender.

Add frozen five-star fruit (carambola) until thick.

## THICK SHAKE

Blend:       16 ounces fresh-squeezed orange juice
1 pint frozen strawberries

Add 1/4 avocado or until thick.

# SERIOUS EATIN'

There are dishes especially for people who want to feel full after their meal. These meals are heavier, richer and tend to look more traditional. I recommend that you save them for special occasions, dinner guests, and holidays.

# ESSENE BREAD

Soak 1 pound whole wheat berries for 24 hours.

Rinse and let sit for 12 to 24 more hours,
rinsing every 6 hours.

Grind soaked wheat to a paste in a food processor,
Champion, or suitable grinder.

Add in 2 tablespoons of powdered dried vegetables.

Form into loaves, patties, balls, etc.

"Bake" loaves on trays in the morning sun, and turn
bottoms up at about mid-day. This bread should be done
by the end of the day in summer. During the winter, dry
bread overnight in the oven, on the lowest setting; with
the oven door ajar about 3 inches.

# VEGGIE NUT HORS D'OEUVRE

Mix:        4 ounces finely ground, soaked nuts
            4 pureed celery stalks
            1 bunch fine-cut broccoli flowerettes
            1 pureed red bell pepper

Add other vegetables to satisfy your taste.

Serve on slices of squash.

## GARBANZO DIP

Sprout 8 ounces of garbanzos and process with the milk of 1 coconut.

Add 1 bunch finely chopped parsley.
A little mint or a few drops of lime are optional.

## CUKE CASHEW SANDWICH

Blend 4 ounces of soaked cashews into cucumber and red bell pepper. Spread on celery stalks or cabbage leaves.

## TABOULI SALAD

Cover 1 pound cracked wheat with 2 quarts of distilled water.

Soak until the wheat is soft (20 minutes to 2 hours).
If all the water is absorbed, add more.

Chop:
- 1 bunch celery
- 2 red bell peppers
- 4 cucumbers
- 1 bunch broccoli
- 1 cauliflower

Mix in chopped vegetables.
Stir in 2 to 3 blended avocados. Serve chilled.

# DRESSING RIGHT

Salad dressings are so easy I am repeatedly amazed at how few people bother to make their own. Most dressings are composed of two main ingredients, something fatty and something with a bite. Traditionally, this means oil and vinegar. I use a nut, seed or avocado for the oily component and any acid fruit for the bite. After that it is simply a matter of using available vegetables and herbs to create the flavor you strive for. Be brave and remember, "for success, dress."

## SWEET RUSSIAN DRESSING

Blend:       3 ripe tomatoes
             1 large red bell pepper
             1 avocado
             Juice one key lime

Mix in 3 finely diced celery stalks.


## SWEET TOMATO WALNUT DRESSING

Blend:       4 ripe tomatoes
             4 ounces of raw walnuts

Add freshly squeezed orange juice to reach the desired consistency .


## CASHEW CUCUMBER DRESSING

Blend:       2 large peeled cucumbers

Blend in soaked cashews to reach the desired consistency.

# TAHINI DRESSING

Blend:    4 ounces raw sesame tahini
3 ounces water
Juice of one whole lemon

Buy raw sesame tahini at your health food store or make it by running raw, hulled sesame seed in the food processor with as little water as possible.

Add water until creamy.

# SUNFLOWER VEGETABLE DRESSING

Blend:    4 ounces sunflower seeds
(soaked, raw, hulled)
4 to 6 ounces of water
Vegetables of your choice
(Broccoli, cauliflower, carrots
celery and/or pepper work well.)

# ORANGE JUICE SPECIAL DRESSING

Run 4 ounces of raw cashews through food processor until fine.

Add fresh-squeezed orange juice to reach the desired consistency.

## COCO LOCO DRESSING

Run all the milk and half the meat of 1 coconut through the food processor until fine.

Add pineapple to reach the desired consistency.

## OPEN SESAME DRESSING

Blend:      4 ounces raw sesame tahini
            Juice of one key lime
            1 sprig of mint
            Water
Add sufficient water to create a creamy dressing.

Optional: add one herb (parsley, oregano, basil, rosemary, cilantro, or arugala) to completely change this dressing.

## TOMATO OLIVE DRESSING

Briefly blend: 4 tomatoes
               24 pitted, whole black olives

## SUNNY'S FAVORITE DRESSING

Run 4 ounces raw sunflower seeds through the food processor with any acid fruit until creamy.

## HERB DRESSING

Blend 2 tomatoes with a sprig of any one of the following fresh herbs; anise, basil, oregano, and rosemary.

Add celery as needed to thicken this mix.

Optional: add in the juice of one lemon.

## CREAMY HERB DRESSING

Blend:     2 tomatoes
1 avocado
1 sprig of one of the following herbs:
- Arugula
- Dill
- Cilantro
- Purslane

For a saltier flavor add celery to taste.

# TROPICAL TREATS

Be on the lookout for foods you have not tried. Whereas simplicity is instrumental to the good digestion of each meal, diversity in your overall diet is essential to ;nsure nutritional sufficiency. Eating new foods usually results in unexpected pleasures. Try items you haven't yet tasted, ask your grocer for assistance. Here are a few of my local favorites.

# GUANABANANA

Fresh guanabana (also called soursop) is a subacid-to-sweet treat eaten throughout the tropics.

Dice 2 bananas into a bowl of deseeded guanabana for a delicious meal.

## CUSTARD'S FIRST STAND

There is a class of fruit called anona, eaten worldwide in warm climates.

These include atemoya, cherimoya, anon, sugar apple, soursop, sweetsop, custard apple, pond apple, rolinea, and many more.

The Mona Lisa Custard Apple is increasingly being cultivated in South Florida.

If you can find it, buy it. Allow it to fully ripen and enjoy it with almost any other fruit.

# I'M IN LOVE WITH ROLINEA

Rolinea is a fruit which, when fully ripe, has the color, texture, consistency, and taste of rice pudding. Enjoy it all by itself for a delightful meal.

# HOW'S YOUR MOM BEEN?

The red mombin plum tree may be the most prolific of all fruit-bearing trees. It yields up to six crops per year, each time literally covering the tree with small, fire-engine-red, delicious plums. The taste is something like pineapple and peach. Enjoy them fresh, or put frozen mombin in a bowl of fresh-squeezed orange juice.

# JAMAICAN CHERRY CRUSH

The Jamaican cherry tree, possibly the fastest-growing woody fruit tree, produces a prodigious quantity of fruit the year round. A small white fruit with tiny internal seeds, the Jamaican cherry taste reminds some of caramel, others of the smell of hot buttered popcorn. Mash a pint of cherries into a bowl with 1 or 2 fully ripe bananas. Delicious.

# Some of Dr. Graham's Products

- *What is a Poison?* - Chart
- *Carbohydrates Explained* - Chart
- *What Science Reveals About Raw Foods* - Chart
- *The Answer to Cancer* - Chart
- *The Facts About Flesh* - Chart
- *The High Energy Diet* Nutritional Chart
- *The Cause of Health* - (10 Audio Cassettes)
- *Sunlight* - Audio
- *Water* - Audio
- *Grain Damage* - Book
- *Nutrition and Athletic Performance* - Book
- *The High Energy Diet Recipe Guide* - Book
- *Nutrition and Athletic Performance* - Video
- *Why Consistency Brings the Best Results* - Video
- *The S.A.D. Truth About High Protein Diets* - Audio
- *The Cause of Health* - Video
- *The High Energy Diet* - Video
- *Simply Delicious Recipes* - Video
- *Essential Habits for Exceptional Health* - Video
- *Graham, Wolfe, Clement Panel* - Double Video
- *Hygienic Fasting* - Booklet
- *The Perpetual Health Calendar*
- *Succeeding Socially with a Raw Food Diet* - CD
- *Optimizing Your Training* - CD
- *How Much Fruit Is Too Much?* - CD
- *FAQs and Fiction About Raw Food* - CD

To order any of the products listed above, call the order department at 305-852-0214. You may securely leave your credit card number on the machine. Be sure to also give your name and shipping address. Visit our Web site at www.DoctorGraham.cc. Send an email to mbgraham@aol.com for prices and product availability.

# About the Author

Dr. Douglas Graham, a twenty year raw fooder himself, is an advisor to world class athletes and trainers from around the globe. He has trained professional and Olympic athletes from many sports, including tennis legend Martina Navratilova, NBA pro basketball player Ronnie Grandison as well as the United States Olympic Diving team, the Norwegian National Bicycling team and many Olympians from Aruba. Models, actors, physicians, performers and motivated people from all walks of life have sought his inspiration and guidance as health coach. Mark Victor Hansen, co-author of the *Chicken Soup for the Soul* series is one of his long term clients.

Dr. Graham is the best-selling author of *The High Energy Diet, Perpetual Health, Nutrition and Athletic Performance* and *Grain Damage*. He has shared his strategies for achieving optimum health with audiences at events sponsored by the American, British and Canadian Natural Hygiene Societies, the North American and the European Vegetarian Societies, the American Vegan Society, Earth-Save International, Fitness Professionals U.K., the American Fruitarian Society, and countless others.

Dr. Graham served on the Board of Governors of the International Association of Professional Natural Hygienists and the Board of Directors of the American Natural Hygiene Society. He is a founder of and is currently serving his second term as President of Healthful Living International, the only international Natural Hygiene organization. He is on the Board of Advisors of Voice for a Viable Future, Living

Light Films and EarthSave International and serves as nutrition advisor for the magazine, Exercise, For Men Only. The raw foods and fitness advisor for VegSource. com, Dr. Graham also teaches the Health Educator program at Hippocrates Institute. For ten years he was the owner and director of Club Hygiene, a fasting retreat in the Florida Keys.

His unique vantage point has allowed him to function as a liaison between the various raw food leaders, helping them all to present a more unified front. Dr. Graham's ability to reach a mainstream audience with a healthy raw food message has brought thousands of people into this movement. Dr. Graham's boundless energy and joy for living is definitely contagious.

A professional speaker since 1980, Dr. Graham seeks to make a point while making a friend. He always congratulates people for what they have achieved and motivates them to strive for more.